E

P F

Z O T

D E L P

D F C E P

P Z C F D E

D Z P O L E F

C E T O P F E D

WHICH LOOKS BETTER, 1 OR 2?

Finding the Answers to 21st Century Vision Care

Tim Fortner

First Printing: Which Looks Better, 1 or 2?
Author: Tim Fortner
© 2016
All rights reserved.

This book or parts thereof may not be reproduced in any form, stored in a retrieval system, or transmitted in any form by any means without prior written permission of the author, except as provided by United States of America copyright law.

Cover Art and Design: Eleos Press
                        www.eleospress.com
Interior Formatting: Eleos Press
                        www.eleospress.com

ISBN-13: 978-1540758903

PRINTED IN THE UNITED STATES OF AMERICA

DEDICATION

*Dedicated to my father,
William Harold Fortner, O.D.
1939 Graduate of
Southern College of Optometry
He led the way and started
the tradition of service.*

*Dedicated to my brother,
William Phillips Fortner, O.D.
1967 Graduate of
Southern College of Optometry
He continued the tradition, built upon it,
and carried it into the 21st century*

*Dedicated to our daughter,
Carrie Fortner Irvine, O.D.
2003 Graduate of
Southern College of Optometry.
She carries the tradition
forward into the future.*

TABLE OF CONTENTS

Introduction i
Chapter 1: The Future Ain't What It Used to Be! 1
Chapter 2: The Challenges 9
Chapter 3: Do You See What We See? 19
Chapter 4: Taking Control of the Conversation with Storytelling 21
Chapter 5: Up-Serving/The Method of Creating Loyalty 33
Chapter 6: The Telephone: Smart Phone Etiquette 35
Chapter 7: Reception: Your Story Begins 41
Chapter 8: Pretesting: Conversational Education Begins Here 47
Chapter 9: The Examination: They Don't Call It a Quiz 53
Chapter 10: The Baton Pass: Passing of Authority .. 63
Chapter 11: Frame & Lens Selection: The 61% Solution 69
Chapter 12: The Delivery 77
Chapter 13: Follow-up 83
Chapter 14: By the Numbers 89
Chapter 15: Up-Serving Communications and Strategies 99
About the Author 127

INTRODUCTION

I have spent almost 50 years in the optical industry, beginning on the mail desk and delivering Rxs to local accounts in the late 1960's while attending college. I first worked for Herman J. Muller in Jackson, TN. Mr. Muller was a friend of my father, William Harold Fortner, who was an optometrist.

After college I worked in the front shop running an AIT edger, learning the business from the older employees who trained us, as most of us did in those days. I am grateful to all those who have helped me learn and shaped my career. In fact, I am still learning to this day. I would soon enter the field of sales and call on eye care professionals in West Tennessee, Kentucky, Mississippi and Arkansas. My education continued as I learned from successful eye care professionals. It is my privilege to share what I have learned from them with you. Hopefully it will not only help you in some small way, but you can also pass it on to others as they begin their journey in one of the most rewarding careers one can enter: vision care.

From the 1960s through the 70s we saw changes in frame styles. Plastic lenses replaced glass and large, oversized designer frames became the rage with fashion tints and short-lived fads like facet lenses. In 1980, following Mr. Muller's death, a new owner, Bob Long came to be my boss and mentor. He brought in a national speaker named Bob Bieber. Bob Bieber inspired me to want to do what he did so well!

Fast forward to 1989, I was now vice president and we had a lab in Tennessee and Florida. We had been very successful in the marketing of Varilux Progressive Lenses and were recognized as the Varilux Distributor of the year. It was at this time we were approached by PPG to test-market a new breakthrough in plastic photochromic technology. It was a prototype of what would become the most successful photochromic brand in the world, Transitions Lenses.

After a successful test-market, I went to work with Transitions, a new startup company in 1990 and over the next 25 years we built a world class company which sold in 2014 valued at 3.4 Billion dollars! I had by that time given more than 1,200 seminars to more than 100,000 eye care professionals on six continents. All the time learning from successful business men and women from around the world.

I know technology will continue to change the way we correct vision. So this book is of a more timeless nature, as it deals with the art of communicating educating. It all begins with a conversation; a particular method I call "conversational education."

And, last, a word of thanks to Peggy Hynes. Peggy and I have worked together since my time with Transitions. And more importantly we have remained friends. Her assistance editing this book has been invaluable!

The most valuable lesson I have learned is when you share what you have learned; you gain the right to learn more.

Thanks to all of you for helping me learn!

-Tim

VISION CARE IN THE 21ˢᵗ CENTURY

Chapter 1: The Future Ain't What It Used To Be!

The above quote is one of Yogi Berra's famous quotes, which makes more sense every day. Almost every area of our lives is changing. Politics are changing. The way we shop is changing. Dollar Shave Club shocked Gillette with its simple plan to take away one less shopping chore for men, by shipping them a razor supply once per month. Uber and Lyft are changing transportation and perhaps revolutionizing car buying forever. Robots will be in every household by 2025, we are told. Going house hunting? Virtual reality allows you to put on their gear, have a seat and tour the homes of your choosing. With Amazon Fire TV, I actually can speak into a small microphone on my remote control: "Movies with Robert Duvall" and a list of his movies pops up. So let's take a look at what is happening and what the future holds.

<u>What's New?</u>
1. New Consumer
2. New Technology
3. New Competition
4. New Delivery System
5. New Aging

<u>New Consumer</u>

The internet has changed everything. It has revolutionized buying and the buyer. The new consumer has gotten better at buying than most sellers are at selling. The internet provides the buyer with information parity. Armed with information, this new consumer calls for a change in the way we offer products and services. They have information, and they aren't afraid to use it! They are easily bored by the same-old, same-old. They love new, innovative, unique, and fascinating. They love their technology because it provides convenience. And they really, really hate inconvenience!

This new consumer is skeptical. They aren't easily impressed. You need to earn their loyalty and their trust. They no longer are that impressed by your white coat. They need you to connect with them: what can you do for them that will improve their lives? And how can you do it so you are seen as innovative and fascinating, not the same-old, same-old?

Think about educating this new consumer. Being in health care, patient education is especially important. Teaching your patients how to enjoy the best vision and eye health are musts. In fact, the most often quoted portion of the Optometric Oath is, "I will fully and honestly advise my patients of all which may serve to restore, maintain and enhance their vision and general health. I will strive consciously to broaden my knowledge and skills so that my patients may benefit from all new and efficacious means to enhance the care of human vision." Continuous learning and constant improvement of skills includes revitalizing your story.

WHICH LOOKS BETTER, 1 OR 2?

In this book you'll find a lot of best practices on teaching your patients something new they need to know to make their lives better. It all begins with a conversation. We will explore how to start a conversation and utilize a technique called, "conversational education."

Here are three questions to ask yourself to help you clarify your teaching message:

1. What do you want them to know?
2. What do you want them to feel?
3. What do you want them to do?
* *To Sell is Human*, Daniel Pink.
   (Riverhead Books, pg. 179)

New Technology

New technology has given us things we didn't know we needed and now can't live without. The smart phone culture has changed our lives and how we communicate more than anything. Of course we call them smart, because they are smarter than we are! Smart phones, laptops, iPads have changed the photography business, the land line telephone, entertainment (visual and audio), the book store business, and have created a compulsive obsessiveness to stay connected all the time to everyone. Mobile marketing is now a must for business!

But this new technology has changed the world of vision also. We are no longer looking at 3 inch black letters on a white screen at 20 feet. We spend most of the day looking at pixels on our lap tops and smart phones. We are fast becoming a near-point society. AOA and Vision Council both recommend part of your teaching message should include: "Every 20 minutes take 20 seconds to focus on something 20 feet away." This avoids fatigue which comes from spending hours looking at pixels which cause eye strain and irritation. New technology in the form of free-form digital lenses provides a new and better way of recreating perfect vision. A prescription is not in the numbers we write pertaining to the correction. A prescription is a detailed plan or program which includes multiple pairs offering the latest technology combined with multi-lens apps.

Make sure all of your patients have an opportunity to upgrade to the latest, newest technology. Seeing their best and looking their best is always the end goal. New technology that will make their lives better will go a long way in building loyalty with these new consumers. It's one of the best tools you have. Use it!

New Competition

The internet has created a global economy which can be surfed via the web. This means you now face global competition. The two most frequently purchased optical products bought on the internet are frames and contact lenses. And you can now get refraction online! These providers make it as easy as possible to do business with them. Over-the-counter reading glasses and plano sunglasses continue to grow also.

WHICH LOOKS BETTER, 1 OR 2?

You may be surprised to know Apple has an app called "Eye Reader" that magnifies small print up to five times. They are after your presbyopia patients. You risk being forgotten or ignored if you cannot break through with a message which educates, enlightens and creates interest.

New Delivery System

The Affordable Health Care Act has brought significant changes in the delivery of health care, including vision care. There is not only the changeover from paper to electronic, there is also a change of focus from eye wear to eye care. And today, it is estimated 70% to 80% of the patients receiving eye care have some type of third-party program via insurance, government, HMOs, managed care or vision plans. However, we will discover third-party programs are not the problem, as much as the patients' perceptions of the programs are the problem. The result is a discounted marketplace which has squeezed margins of profit. The net profit to gross revenues ratio has declined. The "just-give-me-what-comes-with-my-plan" syndrome is changing the economics of vision care. We hear eye care professionals across the country saying "we are working harder this year, just to stay even with where we were last year."

New Aging

In a recent interview in AARP magazine, AARP caught up with actor Michael Douglas who was celebrating his 70th birthday. Michael's father, the legendary, Kirk Douglas is 100 years old. When asked about his age, Michael spoke for many of the oldest Baby Boomers which will turn 70 in 2016. Douglas said: 70 is young-old, 80 is middle-old and 90 is old-old. We are living longer. The latest demographics, census and actuaries reveal a healthy 65-year-old male will live to be 85 years of age. A healthy 65-year-old female will live to be 87.4 years of age. A Review of Optometric Business study stated: "The most important phenomena currently unfolding in the USA is the aging of the huge, baby boom population."

The Baby Boomer, who changed the last half of the 20th century with their youth, vitality and sometimes outrageousness, is at it again. They are now changing the first half of the 21st century with their aging which is anything but traditional.

In 2014, the youngest boomers, born in 1964, celebrated their 50th birthday. This prompted AARP to declare 2014 the "Year of the Boomer." All of a sudden a population which had an average life expectancy of 47 years in 1900 is close to doubling that in the 21st century. Now the fastest growing demographics are over 50, over 55, over 65 and over 85. The population over age 50 represents 36% of our population. Everyone is looking at the products and services this group will need in this period of their life. We know health issues, including their vision, have risen to the top of the list for this most influential group.

WHICH LOOKS BETTER, 1 OR 2?

They need our help like never before. They want to know what to expect; what is natural part of aging, what is not and most of all--now that we have added years of life—*what can you do to add life to their years?*

They want to enjoy a quality of life having been blessed with longevity. "Healthy Aging" includes maintaining healthy eyesight and vision. Teach them what they need to know to maintain healthy vision. Teach them also what you can do to restore what has been lost through the natural aging process and how new technology can enhance their vision and general health.

Kaiser Permanente, who had $60 billion in operating revenue in 2015, is changing the way they deliver health care which includes vision care. Their focus in "how do we create an experience showing care, compassion and respect, and giving you all the medical information you need?" Their new model clinic features a Thrive Bar which will be staffed with experts who give information (education) on issues such as nutrition, exercise, vitamins and diet. (Fast Company Magazine, April 2016).

Chapter 2: The Challenges

From November of 2014 through December of 2015, I did 48 seminars in 48 different cities. My interaction and conversations with scores of eye care professionals and business owners included asking about their major challenges. From these conversations, three challenges emerged as the major obstacles and defined a seminar which I developed as a result. The seminar is entitled: "The Just-Give-Me-What-Comes-With-My-Plan Syndrome": How it has Changed Vision Care in the 21st Century."

Here are the challenges:
1. The Impact of Managed Care
2. A Sluggish Economy
3. An Over-Informed, Over-Stimulated New Consumer Lost in a Global Market

Impact of Managed Care

Today it is estimated 70% to 80% of the patients have some type of third-party program which provides monies toward their vision care and/or materials. With the new Affordable Health Care Act, we can continue to expect more of the same. Professional fees are being flattened. Patients are opting for the least expensive solution to their vision problems rather than the best solution to their vision problems.

The result is a discounted marketplace. Sixty-one percent reported decreased margins of profit. Forty-one percent reported increased costs associated with changes in managed care and the amount of work complying and filing for reimbursements. Private pay patients are few and far between. As a result, we heard the same complaint over and over: "We are working harder this year, just to stay even with where we were last year." One of the dangers is patients becoming loyal to their plan rather than their eye care professional.

The industry data reveals the average practice receives from 61-63% of their revenues from materials: frames, lenses, contact lenses and misc.

The following is a breakdown of market share by the three major groups for revenue and for patients:

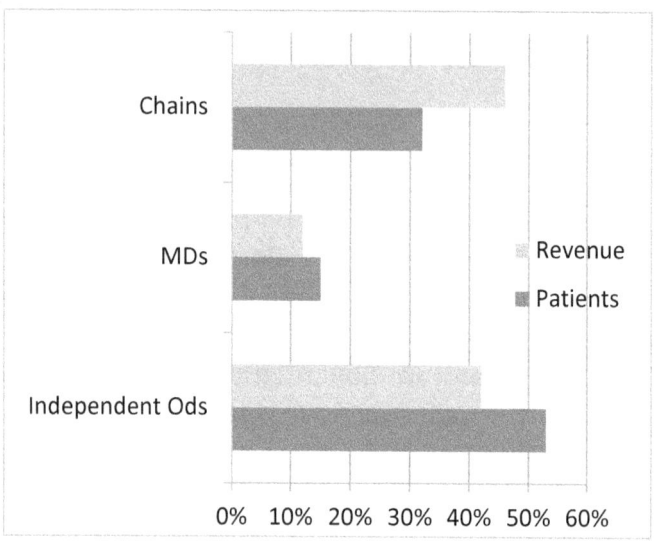

WHICH LOOKS BETTER, 1 OR 2?

These numbers reveal three types of patients:
1. A group which is 100% loyal to their independent provider for both exams and materials.
2. A hybrid group which obtain their exam from their independent ECP and materials from a chain, the internet or a combination of the two.
3. A third group which is 100% loyal to the chain for exam and materials.

The 2nd and 3rd groups are growing at the expense of the first group.

Vision care is a unique health discipline. It is unique in that once the patient leaves the exam room, they become a shopper who is looking not only for a solution to their problem, the function of Rx lenses, but also fashion. They bring with them all their shopping experience plus all the resources they now have online in a global market. People want to see their best and look their best. Educate them how to accomplish this using their third-party program like a Macy's gift card after Christmas. Show them how to get the most value for their money, not just the lowest price.

A Sluggish Economy

This problem magnifies the first problem. We have not only a discounted marketplace; it is taking place during a prolonged period of a sluggish economy stuck at 2% growth. Which means the margin for error is slimmer than ever before. You must take advantage of every patient encounter. Our economy runs on consumer spending: it's 70% of our GDP. In other words, the heart of our economy depends on consumer confidence which drives consumer spending.

Unfortunately, too many patients look at vision care as somewhat discretionary. When money is tight, vision care is postponed. What's frustrating is that the same people who delay their visit to your office because of a sluggish economy don't think twice about upgrading to the next generation smart phone as soon as it becomes available!

Think about this: the average person spends 24 cents per day on primary eye care ($88 per year) while spending $2.77 per day ($1014 per year) on cable television. (Consumer Expenditure Survey: U.S. Labor Bureau)

This brings us to our next challenge—a consumer who is really difficult to engage.

A New Over-Informed, Over-Stimulated Consumer in a Global Shopping Mall

We live in a world that is saturated with communications. Consider the fact we now have 500 channels on our big flat screen televisions plus Netflix which offers up to 70,000 titles and yet we spend our evening surfing the channels via our remote control to find something worth watching. Almost counter intuitive, but as we have more options, we become more easily bored. We live in a world suffering from Attention Deficit Disorder.

WHICH LOOKS BETTER, 1 OR 2?

This consumer is tired of "same-old-same-old." They are intrigued by the new, the unique, the innovative, the fascinating in products, services and information. They love convenience and loathe inconvenience. And, you have to earn their attention.

A recent study and documentary by the BBC concluded the attention span of the average person is that of a goldfish, about nine seconds. I tested this myself by going on Google to get information and found when viewing the hundreds of pages regarding a topic, I only read two sentences to decide if I would open that article or move on to the next. How long did it take me to read two sentences? Approximately nine seconds!

We have to break through to be heard. Between the ever-present ear buds and the ever-present smart phone this is a challenge. This involves strong communication skills, patient education which teaches them something they did not know. It needs to be: innovative, personal and even ***fascinating.***

The following information comes from the well-documented research of the book, "The Challenger Sale." It provides an insight to why this new consumer buys what they buy and whom they buy it from:

Nineteen percent buy based on brand. Brands are not as important as they used to be, but still play an important role.

Nineteen percent buy based on product and service delivery. This says your products and service are adequate and met our expectations. This creates satisfaction. But a satisfied patient will shop anywhere, anytime. Not so with a loyal patient.

Nine percent buy on based on value to price ratio. In other words, I got my money's worth.

This adds up to 47% of the buying decision process. These are must-haves. But the remaining 53% of the buying decision process is where the tipping point is found.

The remaining 53% said it was the purchasing experience itself. Listen how the described the experience:

*Offered unique, valuable perspective of my needs
*Helped me navigate the alternative and avoid pitfalls
*Provided ongoing advice and education
*Educated me about things I did not know, I needed to know
*Educated me about outcomes and what to expect
*Easy to do business with
*Friendly, knowledgeable, helpful team.

This process is the epitome of "enlightened self-interest." The use of conversational education was the key component which made the encounter worthwhile.

Getting and holding the patient's attention is the job of communication, and up-serving, which we address next. To finish our discussion of today's challenges, below are some considerations to position your practice in the face of every expanding managed

WHICH LOOKS BETTER, 1 OR 2?

vision care, a sluggish economy and a consumer always looking for the new, the best, and the shiniest.

Addressing these Challenges Checklist:

- ✓ Do you and your team have regular meetings?
- ✓ Do you have well-thought out answers to frequently asked questions? (Example: why do these costs so much?)
- ✓ How do you keep up with new technology and information?
- ✓ Trade Journals?
- ✓ Seminars/ meetings?
- ✓ Trade shows?
- ✓ Sales reps?
- ✓ Do you and your team wear the latest technology and fashions?
- ✓ Are you aware of your competition's pricing and marketing strategies?
- ✓ Do you have employees in the 50+ age group?
- ✓ Do you offer AARP discounts?
- ✓ Do you have a well-maintained website?
- ✓ Do you do follow-up surveys?
  - o What do you do with information from surveys?
- ✓ In addition to these numerous conversations and exchange of ideas, I would recommend the following books for additional resources and information in dealing with these three challenges. (All available on Amazon).
  - o "The Value-Driven Eye Care Game: A Player's Survival Guide," Larry J.

Alexander, O.D., F.A.A.O. Alistair L. Jackson, M.ED., F.A.A.O. Discusses the role of primary care in this alphabet world of health care programs, plans and insurance.
- "How to Measure and Improve Staff Productivity in Private Practice Optometry," Jerry Hayes, O.D. Discusses how to measure and increase staff productivity, understanding the new economics third-party programs have created.
- "The Challenger Sale: Taking Control of the Customer Conversation," Matthew Dixon and Brent Adamson. Discusses why we buy what we buy and whom we buy it from. These will help you develop conversational education to enlighten the self-interest of your patients

COMMUNICATION IN THE 21st CENTURY

Chapter 3: Do You See What We See?

This book is not about clinical procedures. Industry data shows your expertise and quality of care is highly rated in this area. Nor is it about the science of vision or the new technology of free-form lenses. It is about communication, both written and spoken. It's how we influence others. It's telling the best story and creating a bond of trust with our patients

You cannot make someone listen. But you can entice, inspire, stimulate, and fascinate. Today we have an information overload. Breaking through the clutter to get anyone's attention is a major challenge. Don't forget—a documentary by the BBC likened the attention span of today's consumer to that of a goldfish, approximately nine seconds.

Influence goes beyond grabbing someone's attention and connects to something they already feel is important: themselves! When you can get patients' attention with information about themselves, you will get the goldfish to focus out of self-interest. This book will share some ways to do that—something we call "telling the best story." We have gathered these stories from best practices all around the world.

This is important in terms of grabbing and maintaining a patient's attention. And it's an absolute prerequisite to earning the patient's trust!

Tim Fortner

We live in an affluent society, culture and country. Experts have come to realize affluence breeds boredom. How many evenings have you sat in your recliner surfing via your remote control through 400 channels, plus thousands of options on Netflix to find nothing worth watching? People are tired of the same-old, same-old. Think of all the conversations which have started with someone sharing information from their smart phone exclaiming: "Look at this! You are not going to believe this!"

A corollary to easily bored is impatience. The easily bored consumer when faced with a long line, will leave. Breaking through to this consumer/patient is one of our most difficult challenges. To meet that challenge, we have to become excellent communicators. We have to take control of the conversation and one of the best ways to do that is through storytelling. It is a great way to make your expertise and service relatable to people, and build trust in the process!

Chapter 4: Taking Control of the Conversation with Storytelling

Here is what we want to accomplish: we want to create the conversation your patients will have about their eye care experience with you and your team today when they're sitting at their dinner table tonight. To get this goldfish to take the ear buds out of their ears and listen, to get them to look up from the screen of their smart phone, we must dangle the lure of the new, the innovative or the unique in front of them.

Imagine the end of the day conversation with their family going like this:

> Family member: *"So, what did you do today?"*
> Patient: *"I got my eyes examined."*
> Family member: *"How did that go?"*
> Patient: *"Pretty much the same-old, same-old: which looks better 1 or 2? I am never sure of the right answer. Said wasn't much change and I really didn't need new glasses."*

End of conversation.

Alternatively, your patient could recount some things they learned about their eyes and vision system today which were fascinating. And for the next 10 minutes she talked about the information. What if we asked your last patient what stood out about their experience today? And the patient immediately said, "I have never learned as much about my eyes and vision as I did today. It was totally amazing."

This is what this book is about. It is about capturing the attention of this "goldfish patient." It is about getting them to focus with innovative, personalized and fascinating information about their eyes and vision. We already know how important their vision is to them, but time and money spent on vision care is paltry compared to what they spend on other areas which they consider important in our lives.

We will take you through a cycle of service sharing with you a variety of tools Note how to share the stories and education which fascinate. And how to use the tool of conversational education to execute your oath.

Remember this customer service rule: one negative point of contact negates the next three positive points of contact. It all begins with a conversation. Let's take control of the conversation. Let's give them something to talk about!

The Importance of Storytelling

Today's consumer has gotten better at buying than most sellers are at selling. The internet has given the buyer "information parity," taking one of the traditional advantages away from the seller. What a person really wants is someone they can trust to help them buy what is best for them. They want to have faith in you, especially since they are entrusting something precious to them, their eye sight.

Facts do not necessarily build trust. Data, statistics, technical, and clinical jargon do not create faith in you. But put in the context of a story? That can build trust.

Let's take a look at the six types of stories which will serve you well in becoming the trusted source of expertise and creating loyalty. These are detailed in length in a fascinating book: *The Story Factor: Inspiration, Influence, and Persuasion through the Art of Story Telling,* by Annette Simmons, published by Perseus Books Group.

1. "Who I Am" Story
2. "Why I Am Here" Story
3. "The Vision" Story
4. "Teaching" Story
5. "Values-in-Action" Story
6. "I Know What You Are Thinking" Story

Let's touch briefly on each of these.

The "**Who I Am**" story reveals something personal about yourself and why you chose to become an eye care professional. It may have been your own vision problems, or some other facet of your life which shaped your decision and values. People want to do business with people who are friendly, helpful and knowledgeable. This story lets them see you as a sincere, open and friendly person. And it's a marvelous segue to finding out more about THEM. Remember the goal is to make your practice relevant to THEM! These stories can all be shared through an in-office newsletter given to each patient, which introduces them to your office and all about you and your team.

"I was only in the second grade, when my parents noticed me rubbing my eyes, squinting and sitting close to the television. One day I put on my mother's glasses and could see everything better. As a result they took me to see the optometrist where I was diagnosed with myopia and fit with my first pair of glasses. I remember looking at the tree outside the window of his office and saw for the first time the individual leaves. Those glasses immediately made a difference in my life. I realized later, I wanted to be an optometrist so I could make a difference in people's lives." (First year optometric student @ SCO)

The "***Why I Am Here***" story is about your goals as an eye care professional. They can be summed up in a one sentence statement: "Our goal is to help the most people enjoy the best possible vision for as long as possible by the best possible means." The point is to directly involve the patient's well-being in this story.

"I loved my grandfather. He was fun and could do anything. He had his own business, but more than that, he could make anything with his hands, grow vegetables in his garden, flowers in his yard, raise pigs and chickens and virtually put food on his table he had grown or raised himself. He had lost the vision in one eye when he was younger through an infection which

was not properly treated. Later in his 70's he lost the vision in his one good eye through macular degeneration. His blindness changed him completely, from an independent, robust man to one who had to depend on others. Depression and inactivity led to a nursing home and finally his death. I was convinced, if he had not lost the vision in his one eye due to untreated infection, he might have not become totally blind. This is why I do what I do—to help people see their best for as long as possible." (Optometrist in rural south)

The "**Vision Story**" tells others what is important to you and how it connects to them. The successful practice wants to answer all their patients' questions; allay all their fears and tell them what to expect. Together, as a team, they help each of their patients enjoy a better quality of life by enjoying the best possible vision. Everyone deserves the right to see the best they can see.

"I came from a family of eye care professionals, so I became an eye care professional and entered into the family business. But as I began to work with patients, I encountered those who had lost vision in an eye due to an accident—a flying rock from a lawnmower, a caustic chemical in their eyes at work, or through lack of regular medical care which resulted in loss of vision due to glaucoma or diabetes. I came to hate loss of vision, the way an oncologist hates cancer. My vision was to make sure I understood my patients and their lifestyle so I could make sure I was

doing all I could to prevent loss of vision." (Third Generation ECP)

"Teaching stories" are exactly that: stories, illustrations, real life examples that teach patients something they did not know, something they need to know. It gets their attention. One of our goals in this book is to provide you with some fascinating, attention-getting facts.

"It was my first day of optometry school, and the vice president of the school was telling us what to expect in the next four years. I was taking notes furiously, but it was the story he told at the end, which I did not even write down, which stuck with me all these years. He said, 'let me tell you what you are going to be able to do with your education and skills, you will be able to sell tickets to the "movie of life" showing on the screen of the retina.' I realized then and through the next four years, storytelling was a great educational tool and have used stories I have developed to educate my patients. We have such a great story to tell regarding the amazing gift of sight, but some of us are not very good storytellers." (A life-long learner and storyteller)

"Values-in-action" stories talk about something you and your team did for an individual which changed their life. Having testimonies and real-life stories from your patients can be part of what you can display on your website and/or social media. A patient bulletin board in your office can contain communications and photos of patients and patients' stories which reflect your values in action.

"I designed my new office without a window in the exam room. My goal was to be able to create total darkness, the absence of light. Having a rheostat switch on my light, I was able to control the light from full brightness to being able to dim it to stimulate loss of vision to complete darkness. I told my patients, as I brought the light down to total darkness, my goal was to make sure this does not happen to them. I then told them the greatest health fear people have is loss of vision. Telling a best story is always made more powerful with a compelling illustration." (An enlightened ECP)

"I Know What You Are Thinking" stories let your patient know you realize what their concerns are. Today, with online resources, everyone wonders are they getting the best solution at the best price. You must provide reassurance that you will not recommend anything that is not in the best interest of the patient. It may have to do with their interest in buying eyeglasses or contact lenses online, or elsewhere. Consumers are not sure what the price of good pair of eyeglasses should be. Could you and your team tell a value story which would justify the cost and satisfy the patient? Obviously, when your patient asks for their Rx with their PD, you know exactly what they are thinking.

"When I was a student in optometry school, I never liked having to deal with pricing with the

patient. Yet I discovered in the real world price is always a consideration and on the patient's mind. With managed care and third-party programs, patients tend to choose the least expensive solution rather than the best solution. After several frustrating conversations with patients about why they should buy their eyeglasses here, we decided to get proactive and come up with seven reasons why they should get their eyeglasses here. Those are in a brochure we give to each patient along with a sign in our dispensary which says, 'Beware of bargains when shopping for brain surgery, parachutes and eyeglasses!' It gets their attention and reminds them price is not always the main reason for a decision involving matters of health and safety. We also strengthened our warranties and guarantees." (A proactive professional)

I know what you are thinking: I could never say all of that or find the time.

You don't have to say all of it all the time! But you and your team need to practice weaving these storytelling techniques into your dialogue with patients. And of course not all communication is spoken. Develop an in-house communication to be given to each patient which is all about you, your service, your team and contains your stories. An in-office communication should be provided in your office. This all-important patient education is designed as a pre-exam education and a take-home piece. Education needs to be pre-visit, during the visit and post-visit.

WHICH LOOKS BETTER, 1 OR 2?

Remember, telling the best story is always important. Patients aren't going to make up your story. You create the stories they remember about you and that they tell their friends about you. If you don't provide them with those stories, you and your practice won't be memorable. And if patients don't remember you, how do you expect them to be loyal?

Communication in the 21st Century Checklist:

- ✓ Do you have an in-office newsletter for hand out?
- ✓ Does it contain your team's story (bios) and experience?
- ✓ Does it clearly state your mission?
- ✓ Does your office speak with "one voice?"
- ✓ Does each team member know his/her role in engaging with patients?
- ✓ Do you have stories? Have your staff work on at least one or two stories in each of the categories described above.

UP-SERVING IS THE FUTURE

Chapter 5: Up-Serving/The Method of Creating Loyalty

Up-serving is how you are going to drive your practice/business to the next level. It is understanding that vision care is a team effort.

Up-serving is the opposite of upselling. Of all things consumers say they detest, from convoluted phone menus to the insulting on-hold message, 'your call is very important to us'; nothing is more detestable than upselling.

"Up-serving means doing more for the other person than he/she expects or you initially intended, taking extra steps that transform the mundane interaction into a memorable moment." (*To Sell is Human*, Daniel Pink) Up-serving makes service personal and purposeful.

Up-serving is a strategy which has one goal—to create loyal patients. Loyalty has an economic advantage as we look long term at lifetime value of a loyal patient. Loyal patients are more profitable. Loyal patients are ambassadors for your practice or business and create more referrals. A satisfied patient will shop anywhere, anytime; not so with loyal patients. As we go through the cycle of service and view each touch point we will share with you proven strategies, communications, and programs which build loyalty.

With squeezed margins of profits, a sluggish economy and global competition, you must make the most of every patient encounter.

Viewing the experience through the lenses of the patient's eyes will cause you to rethink what the focus of your activities should be: The only thing which really matters is what kind of experience the patient has when they come in and interact with you and your team.

It all begins with a conversation. So let's talk about what happens in the critical touchpoints of service in your office and business. And I'll warn you, implementing up-serving almost always means updating many aspects of patient interaction. (See our Up-Serving Resources in the Resource section.)

Chapter 6: The Telephone: Smart Phone Etiquette

How you handle the phone has a lot to do with attracting and maintaining new patients. This is usually the first contact a new or potential new patient has with your office. It's also one of the primary means of communication with your established patients.

Here are a couple of scenarios which probably occur with regular frequency:

- *An employee of a company finds your name on the list of vision care providers for their plan. They call your number. The phone rings 10 times with no answer. Or worse, you get a recorded message which states over and over: "your call is very important to us..." They hang up and go to the next name on the list of providers.*

- *A parent discovers her 5-year-old has put something in their eye and is screaming bloody murder. In a panic she calls your office. Your receptionists answer in rapid fire words: "Fortner Eye Clinic, please hold. Click."*

The goal of your phone contact with current and potential patients is to make sure you identify the caller's needs and address them efficiently, professionally and in a pleasing manner. You want the caller to think: "This sounds like a place I would really enjoy patronizing."

Tim Fortner

Let's look at what Best Practices do to turn this all important point of contact into an up-serving moment and opportunity.

The Basics:

1. Always answer within 3-5 rings. "Thank-you for calling Fortner Eye Clinic, this is Gina, how may I help you?" If your volume of calls is such that you need an automated answering system, make your message very simple and straightforward. "If you know your party's extension, please enter it now. Otherwise press 0 and an operator will assist you." People like to talk to live people as soon as possible.
2. Always have a back-up. The person answering the phone is often multitasking. A back-up person must be familiar with scheduling appointments, pricing, insurance, hours, services provided—all the normal questions.
3. Always ask: "Are you experiencing any problems with your vision right now?" A problem could qualify as an emergency and your office should always have time to work in an emergency. In addition, this clearly signals your practice's sincere interest in the patient's well-being.
4. Always ask before putting someone on hold: "May I put you on hold for just a minute? Thank-you." If the wait is more than a minute or two, the call handler must come back and

take the caller's number and call them back at a time convenient for the caller.

5. Always confirm the caller has gotten all the information they needed. "Have I answered all your questions?"
6. Always thank the caller. If a current patient: "We appreciate that you have entrusted your vision care to our office; we look forward to seeing you soon." If a potential patient, a phone shopper, say: "We would love to have the opportunity to provide you and your family with vision care. Would you like to make an appointment today?"

Handling Questions:

- Providing price information is a great opportunity to up-serve: don't assume the caller has any how idea how prices are determined in the optical business. So if a caller wants to know, for instance, what brand of lenses he saw advertised costs, don't simply give him a dollar amount.
- Explain lens prices vary by prescription and material starting at this price for a simple Rx in basic material and going up to this price for a more complex Rx in high performance materials. If you can ascertain if the patient wears single vision or is presbyopic, so you can narrow your response to those categories.
- Don't just tell them what an exam costs, tell them what all is included: blood pressure check, refraction for correction and a variety

of tests to determine the presence of any disease or vision threatening conditions. Always inform the phone shopper of added values such as: warranties, guarantees, free lifetime adjustments and repair.
- A printed list of insurance providers your office accepts needs to be easily accessed for quick reference. Regardless of the questions, once it has been answered, make sure to follow-up with: "Would you care to make an appointment with us today?"

Appointments
- Never forget when a patient calls for an appointment, the goal is for you to accommodate the patient's schedule, not the other way around. Ask the patient's preference: time of day, preferred day, their earliest availability and give them a couple of options. Many successful practices offer one day a week for early evening appointments. Today with an aging population and the explosion of Medicare, you might consider early morning slots for the early riser, the retiree.
- Make certain to note the primary reason for patient's examination and place a note in on calendar and the patient's file.
- Clearly articulate your practice policy re: cancellations once the appointment is set. Set up the best means for reminder of appointment—e-mail; text, phone call. When

contacting by email—you can also attach a pre-visit message to help the patient get the most out of the upcoming appointment and begin the educational process.
- If the patient is looking for an appointment ASAP, obtain their number and tell them, you will call them back to advise them of an opening.
- Once the appointment is set, confirm payment policies; instruct them to bring: all their current prescriptions with them; proof of insurance and also let them know how long their appointment will last.

Up-serving Looks Like This:

1. When making an appointment, ask if there is another family member that is due for an exam; if convenient, suggest one trip for two appointments.
2. The name game: always address the patient by their name. If an adult always use last name with proper prefix—i.e. Mr. Fortner, not Tim. Always identify yourself by name in case the call is interrupted the caller will know who to ask for when calling back. It is frustrating to explain the same issue over again, because you do not have the name of the person you talked with previously.
3. Why is this person calling? They want information. They want to check on something they have ordered. They want to talk to a

particular person – the doctor, the optician, the person who files insurance. They want to buy something from you. If the average revenue generated per examination is $300, then converting one shopper per day to an appointment would be worth $75,000 in gross revenues per year.

Up-serving Doesn't Look Like This:

1. The person who handles that is not here today. (Instead: "The person who handles that is not here today. But if you can tell me what you need, I am sure we can take care of it for you.")
2. We are currently out of stock on that. (Instead: "We are currently out of stock of that item. Do you know the size and color you want? We can order those and have them here in a day or two. I can also email you the size and color information so you can take a look at the choices.")
3. The doctor is busy. (Instead: "The doctor is with a patient now. May I ask if this is an emergency? If not, he/she will be able to call you back between 10:30 and 10:45? Will that work for you? Good. Can I ask the nature of your problem if it is not too personal so the doctor can pull your file? ")

Chapter 7: Reception: Your Story Begins

The impression your office makes on patients when they enter is critical. You want that impression to be inviting. Not just clean—pristine. A great first impression starts the process of a smooth and educational flow through your practice.

Scenarios:

- *Patient enters your office. At the reception area are two employees: One is inputting data in the computer and does not look up. The other is on the phone—she makes eye contact and checks you in by pointing to a sign and lip-synching—"Sign in, please." People in the front office, the reception area, must be champion multitaskers. The employee on the phone then hands the patient a clipboard and tells them: "Fill out the front and back. We will call you when we are ready."*

- *Patient accepts the clipboard and takes a seat and begins to fill out the requested forms. Perhaps wondering, does anyone look at this? The average wait time in a medical practice in the USA is 18-23 minutes past the appointed time, depending on the type of practice. What is going through their mind: "Hey, I'm ready now. I have to be somewhere in an hour—if this going to take longer than that? How much longer?" The feeling they are experiencing is an attitude of indifference by your team to their time and situation. The longer the patient feels ignored and their time is not being treated as important, the more this patient is asking himself: "why am I still coming here?"*

The Basics:

1. Always be mindful of common senses. Sense of smell, sight, touch and hearing. One best practice said they had invested in scent diffusers to provide a pleasant aroma in their office. Retail businesses have known for years: there is a strong connection between the sense of smell and mood. Lighting, decor, cleanliness also creates a pleasant atmosphere. Sometimes you don't see your surroundings in the same way someone walking into your office for the first time would. A water stain of the ceiling. Dust on the blinds. A dead plant in one corner. Old magazines displayed in a haphazard manner. Pleasant sensory experiences have proven to play a role in buying decisions.
2. Always print a list of patients for the day and distribute to the staff. This will enable everyone to greet patients by name. The check-in at the reception starts the process and cycle of service. A great first impression

here starts a smooth and instructive flow through your practice.

3. Always take time to emphasize the importance of the information you are asking them to give. Explain they may have experienced some changes since their last visit and you want to make sure you update their patient profile. Explain the flow to the patient. "You will be seeing Margaret first, she will do those preliminary tests which will get us started and begin the process of gathering some basic information to assess the health of your vision. "

4. Always escort the patient from one area to the next, introducing the patient to the next team member and repeat to the team member why Ms. Hynes is here today. The handoff should include not only the introduction, but also something about this team member's expertise. "You are in good hands with Margaret; she has been doing this for more than 12 years. She is truly an expert. "

The Patient Profile

The Patient Profile begins in the reception area, but it is reviewed by each team member who interacts with the patient, especially the doctor. This information, so often taken for granted as the 'same-old-same-old' information should be updated in order to up-serve. (Remember this: up-serving almost always includes updating)

Tim Fortner

As strange as it sounds to people in our business, most people take their sight for granted. Your job is to help them think about their vision and how the use it. The profile is a key component.

Here are some suggestions of questions to ask to update your patient profile:

At Work:
- Do you perform fine or close-up work?
- How much time do you spend on the computer?
- Are you required to wear safety protection for your eyes?
- Are you outdoors all or part of the day?

Driving:
- Do you have trouble reading signs at night?
- Do you have a long commute to work?
- Do you drive into the sun, coming or going to work?

Lighting:
- Are you bothered by overhead lighting?
- How about computer and other digital lighting?
- Oncoming headlights?
- Have you noticed you are more sensitive to bright sunlight?

General:
- Do you have trouble with small print?
- Do you have trouble with dark adaptation or night vision?
- What hobbies or sports do you enjoy?
- Do you travel a lot for business or pleasure?

WHICH LOOKS BETTER, 1 OR 2?

Keeping this information in the patient's file and having staff review it prior or during their visit gives your team the opportunity to up serve your patients.

The best eye care professional is the one who knows their patients best!

Updated profiles should note significant events—a special trip, a wedding, recent job changes, or lifestyle changes—retirement or semi-retirement.

One of my observations of successful practices is they show a natural curiosity and interest in their patients. They ask good questions, listen, observe and take notes.

Up-serving Looks Like This:

1. Scent diffusers.
2. Patient Appreciation Bowl.
   - Put a crystal bowl on the reception desk with a simple contact form next to it. Label the bowl "Patient Appreciation." Patients filled in their contact info and put it in the bowl. Each Friday, draw a name out of the bowl and award a $50 gift card. The note with the card said in appreciation of your loyalty to our practice. The $2500 spent per year on this simple plan not only created 50 families who were now loyal and cheerleaders, it also helped them update contact -information for their other patients.
3. Updated Patient Profile.

4. Cleanliness. Current newspapers and magazines. Cut the clutter
5. Smooth check in and staying on time gets the experience started in a positive way.
6. Relevant, attention-getting educational materials in reception.

Up-serving Doesn't Look Like This:

1. The odor of reheated Chinese food drifting out of the break room
2. A water stain of the ceiling. Dust on the blinds. A dead plant in one corner.
3. Old magazines displayed in a haphazard manner.
4. Your patient Mrs. Fortner is taken to the empty pre-exam room and sits down to wait for the para-optometric. He walks in a few minutes later: "Are you Mrs. Hynes?"

Chapter 8: Pretesting: Conversational Education Begins Here

Remember what one of your goals is: to change and influence the conversation the patient has tonight with their spouse or significant other regarding their eye examination and interaction with you and your team today.

Do these scenarios sound familiar?

- *Your new patient is wearing eyeglasses. She has NOT been happy with them, that's one reason she came to you instead of the big box chain she had been patronizing. During the pre-exam she waits for the tech to ask about her current eyewear. And waits, and waits…*
- *The para-optometric has the patient position herself for tonometry, casually advising the patient "Ok this puff of air won't hurt." Afterwards he makes some notes and moves on to auto-refraction. That's the extent of the dialogue.*

When asked about their experiences will your patients say: "It was pretty much the same-old, same-old. Which looks better 1 or 2? I am never sure of the right answer. They also said there was very little change in my prescription and everything looked good, so I didn't need any new glasses."

OR when questioned about their eye exam and experience will they launch into some interesting information they learned that day, they did not previously know, but needed to know? Your patients do not make up stories about your practice and their experience—you and your team create those stories. Let's give them something to talk about.

The Basics:

1. Always ask the patient what they like about their current eyewear and what they do not like about current eyewear. If the patient has brought all of their current prescription eyewear, take note of absence of any which might address vision issues. Example: have AR or not? Computer Lenses? Photochromic? Sun wear? Any special pairs for hobbies and activities?
2. Always review the Patient Profile as part of pretesting. This includes medical history, the reason for the appointment, any vision issues and current eyewear. This is why the updated patient profile is a key component. In asking good questions we have gathered very useful information from the patient about work, driving, computer usage, hobbies, as well as uncovering problems such as: reading signs when driving at night, increased sensitivity to bright sunlight, and trouble reading small print.

3. Always engage the patient in conversational education.

The Conversation

- By utilizing the Patient Profile and conversational education, the patient is educated on his need for a multiple system of vision corrections and lens apps to help restore, maintain and enhance their vision and general health.

  As a result, the patient isn't surprised as the doctor and optician recommend multiple eyeglasses to help them function their best and enjoy enhanced vision.

  Here's an example of how this works: in reviewing the family medical history, you note that this 62-year-old female's mother had glaucoma and her father had macular degeneration. You also note her profession, a registered nurse. She is aware of health issues on two levels—family history and a knowledgeable health care professional. She has high blood pressure and currently takes a daily medication for it. Let's begin the conversation:

  "Mrs. Fortner, I see you are in for your annual wellness exams. Let me review with you what tests we will be doing here. I will be performing an auto-refraction which will give the doctor a base line for your Rx. I will also check your blood

pressure and perform one of the preliminary tests for glaucoma. I notice you are taking a medication daily for your high blood pressure."

- Use conversational education to change what is one of the most routine tests in health care offices (blood pressure) into something they will want to talk about at the dinner table tonight!

    "Mrs. Fortner, do you have any idea how extensive your blood vessel network is? By that I mean, if we took all of the blood vessels out of your body and laid them end to end, how far do you think they would reach?" "I have no idea," she replies. "Would you believe they would stretch 60,000 miles?! What is also incredible, is when we gain 16 ounces of fat, not muscle, our body has to create an additional 7 miles of blood vessels just to service those 16 ounces. High blood pressure, not controlled or treated can also impact your vision. A condition called hypertensive retinopathy."

    All of a sudden, you have successfully broken through the "same old, same old" conversation to an attention-getting fact—which is fascinating!

WHICH LOOKS BETTER, 1 OR 2?

Now as this tech begins to perform the glaucoma test, she educates the patient on what this instrument is and what it does.

> *"Mrs. Fortner at your age and with your family history, a mother who had glaucoma and a father who suffered from macular degeneration, and with your health issues, you need to have these tests done every 12 months."*

- Notice the personalization: <u>your</u> age; <u>your</u> family history, <u>your</u> health issues. The patient has been given very important information they needed to know. And it was based on their age, family history, and health issues. Use that information to personalize your conversation! Best Practices tell us 12 months is more effective than annually or one year.

Up-serving Looks Like This:

1. Use of the Patient Profile can be enhanced by providing educational scripts for your team. These scripts would be designed to educate and enlighten the patient and use those words which are most effective. Avoid clinical jargon and words which can confuse or introduce the wrong idea.
2. A checklist with possible solutions for each area of the patient's profile, where the questions uncovered an issue they were experiencing. For example: do they have trouble reading signs at night? Recommend

AR Coating and explain how, as one ages, changes in the eye cause less light to be reaching the retina. On average, a 60-year-old has approximately one-third of the light entering their eyes as in a 20-year-old. By introducing this idea early in the cycle of service the patient is being prepared educationally why and how this would improve their vision. Same thing with photochromics and polarized sun wear if the profile uncovers light sensitivity, or computer glasses if symptoms of CVS are identified.

Up-serving Doesn't Look Like This:

Use of jargon that has no meaning to the patient. If you use the term "presbyopia," explain what it means—and in a personalized way!

The patient has noted vision issues on the profile, e.g., difficulty driving at night. The pre-tester doesn't ask about it and the patient doesn't volunteer.

Using the term "covers" in relationship to insurance. Best Practices say "contributes." "Covers" implies the cost is completely paid for except for basic co-pay.

Chapter 9: The Examination: They Don't Call It a Quiz

This is why patients come to you; this is where you can leverage the trust they have in your clinical abilities to ensure the patient walks out of your practice more educated and more fascinated with vision, and with the best eye wear solution!

Scenario:

- *Doctor finishes a series of tests, which include a refraction and begins to summarize the findings for the patient:*
    > *"Everything looks good in the back of your eye. No signs of any disease or damage. Your pressures are all in a good range. And there has been very little change in your prescription. Keep doing what you are doing and we will schedule you for your annual wellness exam this time next year."*

How much change is really a '"little change" in today's world of new digital lens technology? Usually this description of "little change" refers to a change of a $1/12^{th}$ of a diopter or less. What was the ECP comparing to when he said there has been little change? When we consider with new free-form lenses we can fabricate a personalized Rx within $1/100^{th}$ of a diopter, this is not a little change!

When asked where they received their last eye exam at a leading school of optometry, the school was shocked to discover one of the most popular answers was when they took their drivers' license test. The vision screening at most drivers' license test consists of asking which looks better, or can you read the letters on this line. Similar language and tests in the doctor's examination make the consumer think they have had their vision tested when in fact they have had only a gross screening.

The Basics:

1. Don't fall into the trap of thinking that recommending the best product solutions is "selling." As a clinician and medical professional your expertise is not questioned. However, as the owner of a small business that derives more than 60% of its revenues from selling products, you probably have little formal training in running a retail business. And one has to be honest about their strengths and weaknesses. But let's take a look at how your clinical strength can strengthen your retail business. There is a way you can grow your business, be innovative, and maintain your professional standards. You can do it and not compromise your ethics, but in fact execute your oath even better and take vision care to the next level by up-serving your

patients. Let us just substitute the word "sell" with "prescribe" and/or "advise." After all, your oath said you would "fully and honestly ADVISE your patients of all that would serve to restore, maintain and enhance their vision and general health." Tell – don't sell.

2. Always connect the back of the eye exam to the front of the eye solution. Frankly, you will never maximize the revenue of your practice without leveraging your clinical expertise to guide your patient recommendations. This calls for you to connect the back of the eye exam with the front of the eye solution. And combining these two is not contrary to your oath—it is, in fact, executing your oath to the best of your ability and knowledge.

3. Always use the patient profile update and checklist your team has been compiling through the cycle of service. Your team has helped you prepare for this moment by utilizing the patient profile update and documenting through the cycle of service. You can see exactly what issues the patient is experiencing. Your clinical, scientific and medical background can educate the patient as to what are the causes of these problems. But it must not end there, having uncovered the problems: you must recommend the solutions which will go in front of the eye to compensate and correct the problems in the back of the eye.

Prescribing a Personalized Prescription Plan for Each Patient:

- Here is a great example of summarizing the exam and other information for a patient: all personalized to ensure the patient continues to enjoy good vision and health and see her best. First summarize the exam results (back of the eye):

    "Mrs. Fortner I am now looking at the back of our eye at the macula of your retina. This is where your father lost his central vision. Everything looks good, but at your age and with your family history, you need to have this test done every 12 months."

    (This is not only wise, prudent and indicated as necessary, it also shortens the cycle of service. Shortening the cycle of service is one of the ways we increase revenues, not by seeing more patients but by seeing our patients more often, especially in this age group. This is up-serving not up-selling. The pre-appointing message has now been repeated and reinforced)

    "Mrs. Fortner, there have been some changes in your vision. We

are going to have to do some things differently. Fortunately there is new technology which will allow us to address these changes better than ever before."

"Let's evaluate what our diagnostic tests revealed today. You have problems with reading signs at night, poor night vision and trouble adapting to dark. We have ruled out through our tests there is no disease causing this problem. These changes are a natural part of the aging process. What makes your situation worse is without AR coating, you are losing up to 14% of the light entering your eyes through lens reflections. Let me explain what is happening, and feel free to interrupt me if you have a question. "

- Always explain what this means to the patient and what the likely problems are—or will be.

   "From now on you will experience problems with small print, low light, night vision, dark adaptation and bright sunlight. You will have a higher incidence of floaters and dry-eye, especially with your computer and other digital devices

you use each day. High blood pressure, which you already have, is common at your age, but must be controlled. You also are at risk for glaucoma, which your mother had. Glaucoma is the second leading cause of blindness among working age Americans. It also has no warning signs, so we strongly recommend regular maintenance examinations. By age 60, you only have one-third of the light entering your eye as you did when you were 20. This is why we recommend AR coating, a lens app which increases the amount of light reaching the back of your eye. You are also at risk for diabetes which is epidemic today. It is the leading cause of blindness in working age Americans. By age 65, usually cataracts are developing. And by age 75, unfortunately, 30% of our senior citizens are at risk for macular degeneration which is the leading cause of blindness in our senior citizens."

- Then, prescribe your solution—front of the eye.
  "For these reasons I am recommending the following plan of treatment to

WHICH LOOKS BETTER, 1 OR 2?

restore, maintain and enhance your vision and general health.

New free-form technology will provide you with the most personalized lenses possible. They will provide you with high-definition vision. I will prescribe two lens apps which will make these lenses in your primary pair of glasses even more versatile. AR coating will allow more light to come into your eyes added with the application of photochromic technology which automatically darkens in bright sunlight. These two new improved technologies will address your issues with not enough light and too much bright sunlight. They will appear as clear lenses indoors and at night, but are activated by the UV of sunlight. These will help enhance your vision in those light conditions.

Your plano polarized lenses worn over your contact lenses is a great solution. You might want to consider a pair of polarized prescription sunglasses for those extended periods of time in the sun or working outdoors. What you wear outside during the day impacts how well you adapt to dark at night.

I will also write a prescription for a pair of computer lenses. The amount of time you are spending on digital devices is putting your vision at risk in the long term due to the blue light exposure being emitted from your digital devices. And I strongly recommend, you remember to take 20 seconds every 20 minutes to look at something 20 feet away to rest your eyes.

Do you have any questions for me? If not—our next step is very important. Our technician will come in to take some very precise measurement for the new digital lens technology. Our team will show you how to maximize your insurance. As always, we will work with your budget—including some alternative ways of obtaining what will best take care of your problems.

Up-serving Looks Like This:

1. You make a specific recommendation, or prescription. Patients, especially those 50 and older, are looking for a trusted source of expertise. Research data shows there is a big disconnect between what patients want from their eye doctor (70% want a lens recommendation) and they actually get (36% report their eye doctor does a great job making a

personalized recommendation). What an opportunity to differentiate your practice from the competition! What an opportunity to up-serve your patients.
2. Providing discounts on multiple purchases and offering alternative financing options
3. Providing your patients with educational materials regarding: vitamins, nutrition, losing weight, quit smoking, UV and Blue Light protection.

Up-serving Doesn't Look Like This:

1. Being unprepared for commonly asked questions. Make a list of the most frequently asked questions and objections. Then sit down with your team and come up with well-thought out answers to these tough questions that everyone is comfortable with.
2. Having confusing warranties and guarantees. Forget the fine print approach:
   - Offer 24-month replace or repair warranties on frames and lenses.
   - Offer free lifetime repair.
   - Consider something really unique, like: a 14-day trial period for new lenses and frames. If during that period for any reason they do not like their glasses they can bring them back and you will replace them with a new pair in the same price range at no costs!

- Strong warranties and guarantees reduce risk and increase the patient's interest.

Chapter 10: The Baton Pass: Passing of Authority

The goal of the baton pass is simple: legitimize the optician as the professional who can fill the doctor's prescription and guide the patient through a well-articulated decision making process. This is a critical point of service and we must remember: more than 60% of revenues come from the optical dispensary.

Scenario:

- *Patient has decided beforehand they are going to take their Rx to the mall, where they saw a really cool pair of glasses they want. Or perhaps they are going to the internet to try a resource one of their friends at work has used and really saved some money. Not wanting to tell the optician what they are planning. They look at their watch and tell them, "I don't have time to do this today, I will be back later."*

What can you do when this occurs? How do you prevent it? Remember: you cannot squander a single point of contact in this competitive marketplace. This point of contact is critical. Everything has been leading up to this. All of your work to this point has been to design the best solutions to the patient's vision problems and concerns. Should not the person who diagnosed the problems also be the one to best solve the problems? This should be your thinking and philosophy.

Here is what the data shows us: independent OD's have 53% of the exams, but only 42% of the revenues. Average capture rate is 68%. How does this impact the bottom line?

The Basics:

1. Always track your capture rate. The average for an independent practice is 68%. The formula is simple: divide the number of patients who bought eyewear at your practice by the number of exams for that same time period. Set a goal of one more pair of eyewear per day through up-serving and conversational education that breaks through and gets the patient's attention? This could impact your gross revenues by more than $85,000 per year, without seeing additional patients. (This is the equivalent revenue created by seeing an additional 283 patients!)
2. Always introduce your optician or tech who will be working to fill the prescription to the patient. Ideally, have the tech come into the exam room and begin the handoff:

    "Mrs. Fortner has shared that she has trouble reading signs when driving at night. She is not pleased with her vision at night. She has also stated she has noticed she is more sensitive in

WHICH LOOKS BETTER, 1 OR 2?

bright sunlight. She likes to spend time outdoors gardening, so I am making the following recommendations for her in her primary pair of glasses: we want to provide her with AR coating to let her see better when driving at night, while adding a photochromic filter which will darken automatically in the bright sunlight and protect her from harmful UV."

"I am also recommending a pair of prescription polarized sun wear for extended periods in sunlight which will help preserve her night vision."

"She needs her add power increased for small print; I am recommending a special pair of computer lenses to help her with the time she spends on her laptop, iPad and smart phone to further protect her from over exposure to harmful blue light."

3. Always reinforce when the patient needs to see you again. The Importance of Brands:
- Prescribe specific brand name products. Best Practices do this for the same reason you prescribe specific brand name antibiotics or eye drops, because you know they will get the best results.
- For that patient who is thinking about going elsewhere, the optician needs to have a comparison list of prices charged for the same

brand name products at other offices. This would require some mystery shopping, but like Progressive Insurance you can show how your prices compare with comparable businesses. Key: always compare to other practices or businesses like yours, not the superstore which sells televisions, groceries, tires and clothing! That's not your competition.

Up-serving Looks Like This:

1. Writing multiple Rxs AND explaining to the patient the purpose for each Rx.
2. Provide take home information for post education of the patient regarding their conditions, and any areas of concern which need to be followed closely. If questions regarding price come up at this time regarding insurance and costs, tell them your team will go over what their insurance provides plus any discounts provided as well as alternative means of financing.
3. Positioning the optician as the expert who has the knowledge, skills and expertise to design the best solutions for the patient's vision problems. The baton pass has to be flawless, for a dropped baton at the exchange is a loss for everyone—patient and ECP team.

WHICH LOOKS BETTER, 1 OR 2?

Up-serving Doesn't Look Like This:

1. Reviewing the recommendation publicly without respecting the patient's privacy.
2. Being hesitant in recommending the best solution—apologizing for the added cost instead of stressing the value of the benefit.

Chapter 11: Frame & Lens Selection: The 61% Solution

With 61% of the revenues in the average practice coming from the sale of materials in the dispensary, this is where future growth will come from in the world of third-party programs and managed care. The most profitable thing one can do is sell a second pair of glasses to the same patient.

These scenarios sound familiar?

- *Patient is escorted to dispensary, but the optician is busy with a patient. The optician tells her, "Someone will be with you in a minute." What does the patient do? Begins to look and try on frames. Finds an expensive designer frame they love and now want. This is not necessarily a problem, unless this means the patient will now scrimp on the lens product in order to have the frame they want. Or the patient's prescription will not work with this frame, creating disappointment.*
- *The patient has been dilated and now cannot see clearly to select a frame and will come back later. This irritates the patient, one more trip he has to make!*

Here is the goal of the dispensary: to integrate and connect the clinical part of the visit with the shopping experience of selecting eye wear. The lens product is where it all begins. The lens products are the connection! Remember this area of the average practice accounts for 61% of the revenues. It is important and it requires your team to be able to accomplish this in a short period of time, while not rushing the patient. This is why the system must be as flawless as possible. Your team must be aware of all new technology; have knowledge of optics, as well as the art and science of frame selection and fitting, insurance, work with patients' budgets, while combining function and fashion. Certainly a daunting task.

The Basics:

1. Always stick to a well-thought-out plan. Having a brochure which familiarizes the patient with lens technology is important. If the optician cannot immediately begin working with the patient, having them read about the different types of lens technology, coatings and materials is a good start.
2. Always look at Patient Profile Update. Ask the patient who is currently wearing eyeglasses, what did they like about their current eyewear? What did they dislike about their current eyewear? This will provide some guidelines. Some offices have an optician who does nothing but the lenses: education,

measurements, writing up Rx, etc. Then have a frame stylist who works now with the Rx and the patient to provide the fashion component: face shape, colors, etc. This can also keep the flow in the dispensary from bottlenecking.
3. Always talk lenses first. You provide medical care in prescribing lenses, that's the priority and most important part of the patient experience.
4. Always take control of the conversation regarding insurance. Never use the word, "covers" in the same sentence with "insurance" but, rather, use the words, "provides" or "contributes." Present this information in a positive way: "Your plan contributes to your costs today for your eye care exams as well as your eyeglasses and materials, which will enable you to get the best solutions for less money."

Team Training and Education

- The opticians or techs who work in the dispensary have a very challenging job. They must be experts in technology, lenses, lens treatments, and availability. They must have a working knowledge of third-party programs, vison plans, managed care and insurance. Add to that combining function and fashion with knowledge of face shapes, colors and styles all in a limited amount of time and you begin to realize how challenging this important area is

to your business and practice. This is why team effort is needed to bring us to this point.
- In addition they must have well-thought out answers for frequently asked questions, such as why are these lenses so expensive? Why shouldn't I go online to buy my frames, contact lenses, etc.?
- These professionals need training and education on a regular basis. It's important to frequently review how your office receives training—is it delivered effectively, in a timely fashion? Do you stress the importance of education?

Up-serving Looks Like This:

1. When a patient is to be dilated, and this is known beforehand: have the patient spend some time prior to the exam picking out three or four frames. And if it is unexpected, offer the patient this option prior to the dilation, if possible. Patients will appreciate your consideration of their time!
2. Use an iPad to capture photos of patients in different frames so patients can view themselves without the aid of their Rx. They can even share the photos with family or friends!

Up-serving Doesn't Look Like This:

1. The doctor has recommended photochromics. And the optician explains the benefits of the

WHICH LOOKS BETTER, 1 OR 2?

lenses. The patient asks if anyone in the office wears them. Nobody does.

2. The doctor has recommended more than one premium lens treatment. The optician explains the features and benefits of each premium individually instead of telling a story around the combined benefits of digitally designed progressives with blue light and antiglare protection.

LENSES AND FRAME CHECKLIST

The dispensary is an area that can turn chaotic in busy times. Patients do not want to feel rushed or hurried in this decision of the process. This is why a well-defined system must be in place from start to finish.

There are a lot of variables here we must consider:
- ✓ Number of exam rooms and doctors: adequate for number of patients?
- ✓ Number of employees assigned to dispensary: adequate to provide personalized, quality care?
- ✓ Do you have a bottleneck in the dispensary at times?
- ✓ Do you have "floaters" who are cross-trained to work in different areas when needed?
- ✓ Do we have enough employees? Dr. Jerry Hayes recommends the ratio of one employee for every $150,000 of revenues.
- ✓ Is there additional equipment you need?
- ✓ Do you need to change or extend your office hours? (Flex schedules?)
- ✓ Does your dispensary have lens demonstration devices? A "Lens App" station?

Tim Fortner

- ✓ Check out your dispensary mirror and look at yourself. Is it positioned comfortably? Do you have a handheld mirror available to easily view frame from the side?
- ✓ Is lighting adequate and flattering?
- ✓ Is there an area of privacy to discuss pricing and what their insurance provides?
- ✓ Do you use an iPad to capture photos of patients who cannot see clearly without their Rx?

Chapter 12: The Delivery

The goal of the delivery and dispensing of a new pair of glasses is not only to make sure the fit is comfortable and the patient is seeing properly, it is also to reinforce the value of the service and products your practice has provided.

For these reasons, the delivery and conversational education which take place here are very important contact points. This is also patient loyalty building time.

Do these things happen in your practice?

- *You've told the patient she can pick up her new glasses on Friday. You get a call Wednesday from your lab that the Rx is giving them trouble. Nobody alerts the patient to a possible delay. She shows up Friday, no glasses.*
- *The lens education brochures that were delivered to your office and explain product benefits and care are never unwrapped; they're gathering dust in the break room.*

Have you ever watched a patient who has just picked up their new pair of glasses from your office? If you could, here is what you would see. The first thing she or he will do when they get in the car is to turn the rearview mirror and look at themselves in their new eyeglasses.

They might then look at any information given to them about these new lenses as well as their bill. What is your patient thinking at this moment? Did I get a good deal? Did I pay too much? Do I really need these? All of these questions should have been addressed previously. But here in the delivery process, be sure to restate the value they are receiving.

Over the next couple of days, your patient will be more aware of ads for inexpensive eyeglasses. Someone at work may be bragging about a new pair of glasses they got online and how much money they saved.

The Basics:

1. Always present the new eyeglasses to the patient with some showmanship: open the case (a nice case is imperative—don't scrimp here) and present the eyeglasses as a jeweler would a piece of jewelry.
2. Always position the eyeglasses for the patient. A standard adjustment should have been made when the glasses came in from the lab. Now a refining of that adjustment makes sure the patient is comfortable—behind the ear, on the nose, etc. Then have the patient look in the mirror.
3. Always review the features and benefits and tie them back into the doctor's recommendation and their specific needs— vocational, recreational, and fashion. Point

out the multi-apps which provide multiple benefits. AR coating, guaranteed scratch resistant coating, a built-warin UV filter (or blue light filter) and photochromics. Like a smart phone it has multiple apps which enhance the performance.
4. Always provide the patient with all warranties, guarantees and any special instructions for care and cleaning.
5. Always provide the patient with a copy of their Rx.
6. Always provide them with your personal business card. Tell them you would appreciate it if anyone asks where they got their eyewear, they would give them your name.

Pre-appointing

- We discussed previously in pretesting and in the exam how the team has spoken with one voice concerning regular maintenance care to keep our patients seeing their best. The doctor's last message to the patient is that due to specific conditions--age, family history, occupation, etc. -- she should have these tests done every 12 months.
- Escort the patient to the reception area for any final payments and make sure the patient is reminded of their next appointment in 12 months.
- Make sure you have all contact information and their preference: email, text, regular mail

Up-serving Looks Like This:

1. Offer to clean the patient's "old" glasses, the ones that they'll probably use for back-up.
2. Make certain to remind patients that adjustments are part of your service; you don't want them to look, or see, anything other than their best!

Up-serving Doesn't Look Like This:

1. The patient picks up his or her new eye wear, tries them on and leaves without hearing a "thank-you."
2. The patient is unhappy with the fit of their new glasses. The optician/dispenser is visibly annoyed and suggests that the patient will "get used to it."

DELIVERY CHECKLIST:

- ✓ Do you review all warranties and guarantees with each patient?
- ✓ Do you have any special warranties? One practice offers a 14 -day Return Policy. If for any reason during the first 14-days they are dissatisfied with their eyeglasses, bring them back and they will make a new pair in the same price range at no extra costs. This may sound like you are asking for trouble. But practices who have implemented this say, "It reduces risk," which increases interest and is excellent for 2nd or 3rd pairs.
- ✓ Are eyeglasses cleaned and in a great case with a cleaning cloth?
- ✓ Do you review all features and benefits?
- ✓ Do you educate about cleaning and care?
- ✓ Shop your competition at the mall and see what they are doing and saying.

Chapter 13: Follow-up

Follow-up is an important part of communications and also education. Our goal is to educate the patient: pre-visit, during the visit in-office, and post visit.

Some scenarios to think about:
- *While surfing the net, your patient comes across an online glasses' website. He bookmarks it for future reference.*
- *Your patient gets lots of compliments from friends on his great new glasses. It doesn't occur to him to recommend your practice to these people.*

My first boss in the optical industry was Herman Muller. Mr. Muller was the consummate sales professional. He always had us send an advance card confirming our regular upcoming visit to our accounts. The card contained a checklist for the office, to remind them of small items they may need which are often overlooked: different types of screws, temple covers, cases, etc. We also sent a thank-you note to each office after the visit for their orders and their continued business. Are you not only preparing your patient pre-visit, are you also following up after?

The Basics:

1. Always send each patient a "thank-you" note within 72 hours. A card personally signed by doctor and hand addressed will likely be opened.
2. Always stay in touch with your patients between appointments. If the average time in-between visits or appointments is more than two years, this means the patient does not hear from you in more than 730 days, while possible receiving numerous messages via advertising, television, radio, billboards and direct mail and email from other vision care providers. Wouldn't it be wise and prudent to stay in touch with your patients more often than a post card recall which states, "Our records indicate it is time for your annual eye exam?"
3. Always segment your patients by age, conditions, activities and interests. Conditions such as diabetes, glaucoma, macular degeneration and hypertension should receive regular updates about new developments in the treatment of these conditions.

The Forgotten Patient

- Another area of needed contact is what I call the "forgotten patient." This is a patient who has not been in for an eye health exam in more than three years. Working your files

WHICH LOOKS BETTER, 1 OR 2?

alphabetically, look to pull anyone who has not been in for their eye health exam in more than three years. We have a sample "re-activation letter" which you can adapt in our communications section. By just pulling two records per day, you can contact more than 40 patients who have not been in for whatever reason in more than three years.

Up-serving Looks Like This:

1. Keep your website fresh and update with news that would interest your patients. Text or email your patient whenever something new that aligns with their interests is posted.
2. Reward patients who send you referrals. A $5 Starbucks' card with a thank-you note will build loyalty!
3. Not pre-appointed? Send a reminder three months before you should see them again. Then again in another three months. A lot of people rely on these reminders to schedule heath care exams.

Up-serving Doesn't Look Like This:

1. Your website is the same today as it was when you first put it up years ago.
2. Is your website optimized for tablets and phones? If you don't know, it probably isn't!
3. You offer discounts to AARP members or military. You don't promote this.

RESOURCES

Chapter 14: By the Numbers

We have thus far established the challenges you face in the 21st century: achieving strong profitable growth in a discounted marketplace, third-party programs have created. Made more challenging by a sluggish economy stuck at 2% annual growth, with the internet creating a savvy consumer with more choices than ever before as to where to buy products.

Managed care accounts for 70-80% of your patient flow and revenues. Your largest checks per month come from these programs. How you and your team manage managed care will determine the profitability of your business.

When considering joining a plan, one must take note of several areas:

1. Will reimbursements cover your chair costs?
2. Does the plan have a history of timely reimbursements?
3. Do you have to use a specific laboratory?
4. How many members are in your specific market area?
5. How does a patient/member of the plan receive authorization?
6. How many providers in your market area are signed up as panel members?
7. Does the plan market or advertise to consumers?
8. Are the plans easy to comply with?

9. Does this plan include Rx fulfillment at your office?
10. List the pros and cons and discuss with your team and fellow ECPs.

Obviously, you need to know your numbers and relevant data to help you make wise decisions. This is the business data which drives your revenues. I love MapQuest driving directions. I have trouble with hearing the instructions on a GPS – so I like written directions.

First thing MapQuest asks is, "Where are you starting?" Then, "Where are you going?"

First thing you must do is know where you are starting. These numbers will be your baseline, your starting point. By comparing to national benchmarks, you can see where you are average, below average or above average. You can then set your goal as to where you want to go from where you are.

There are also many fine consultants who can guide you through the process of how to grow. To increase revenues consider the following areas:
1. Increasing your capture rate.
2. Increasing your revenues per patient.
3. Increasing the number of patient seen per day.

<u>Increasing your capture rate</u> starts with measuring how many of your examinations result in purchase of materials at your office. This involves many factors. Does the patient believe they have a good choice of products in your dispensary both in fashion and price range? Do you have in place strong warranties and guarantees? Do you offer any

discounts for multiple pairs? Do you carry the latest styles and fashions? Do you have a lens app section which educates the patient about AR Coating, photochromics, high-index, polycarbonate, and polarized sun wear?

<u>To increase your revenues per patient</u>, there are many lens treatments or as one best practice calls them, "lens apps." Remember: you are to educate and inform your patient of all that will restore, maintain and enhance their vision. Writing detailed Rxs for multiple pairs is a must to increase your average sale per patient. Increasing revenues per patient can be done in materials, multiple Rxs per patient, or increased medical fees. You need to be sure you have the appropriate number of staff members and/or the proper equipment to perform certain medical procedures.

<u>Increasing the number of patients</u> you see each day involves having the room and space to accommodate an increased flow of patients. Then increasing primary care comes down to delegating certain procedures to staff who are trained in those processes.

The following benchmarks will have changed by the time this book is published, but they are current enough (2014-15) to give us a good idea of some very important areas to measure in your practice/business.

Review these benchmarks and note your baseline. Then consider with your team where you want to go. Small increases in specific areas are the best way to start. You have some very good resources in your lab partners and manufacturers who can help you get to where you want to go.

In his book, *Good to Great*, Jim Collins explains three questions you must ask about your business:

1. What do you do best?
2. What is your passion?
3. What drives your economic engine?

When you discover how to get paid for what you love the most and are the best at—you have found the secret of going from good to great. It is serving your patients with service which is personal, purposeful and delivered with passion. It will set you apart from the others.

Also finding the path to great from good involves learning these four truths:

1. Lead with questions, not answers.
2. Engage in dialogue, not debate, not coercion.
3. Conduct autopsies of what failed, without blame.
4. Build red flag mechanisms which allow you to be aware of problems early.

UP-Serving Tip: Put your best people on your biggest opportunity, not just your biggest problems.

WHICH LOOKS BETTER, 1 OR 2?

BENCHMARKS

The following benchmarks and data come from the MBA Practice Profile. They are based on one optometrist working full time. Many of these categories will show the median, the highest 20% and the lowest 20%.

Average gross per exam

Median Gross	$306
Highest 20%	$416-500
Lowest 20%	$159-251

Complete eye exams per hour

Median	1.10
Highest 20%	1.65-2.18
Lowest 20%	.50-.84

Average capture rate

68% of lenses
64% of frames
76% of contact lenses
DO THE MATH!

> 1.01 exams per hour = 9 exams per day; 45 exams per week.
> - 45 exams X $306 = $ 13,770 per week. Capture rate of 68% = 30 had Rxs filled; 15 had examinations only.
> - The 15 exams only @ average of $70 = $1050
>
> Subtract from the total of $13,770 and you will get $12,720. Which means the 30 patient who had an Rx filled spent an average of $424.
>
> By converting one more patient per day through up-serving methods, you will increase daily average by $354.
>
> This would represent an increase in gross revenues if you did one more Rx per day of $1770 per week or $88, 500 per year. This represents is the equivalent of seeing 290 more patients per year!

Sources of revenue

61%	Product sales (43% Rx eyewear, 16% contact lenses, 2% misc.)
39%	Professional fees (22% eye exams, 17% medical fees)

(We expect to see professional fees continue to be flattened under the Affordable Health Care Act and changes in Medicare reimbursements, making Rx fulfillment more important than ever!)

WHICH LOOKS BETTER, 1 OR 2?

Average markups

Frames	2.6 times
Lenses	2.75 to 3.19 times

(Keep in mind with lower cost materials, the mark up formula may be higher. With higher cost materials, the mark up may be lower.)

Frame mix by retail price points

23%	$100-149
31%	$150-199
23%	$200-299
8%	$300-399
4%	$400 and above

(Here is the rule of thumb: the average selling prices of your frames will be at the midpoint between your lowest priced frame and your highest price frame. If your lowest price frame is $100 and your highest priced frame is $400, your average selling price will be approximately $250. Putting in a limited collection of higher priced frames will increase your average selling price.)

Eyewear dispensed per 100 exams

Median	61 pairs
High	109 pairs
Low	49 pairs

Progressive lenses dispensed

Median	65%
Highest 20%	80-90%
Lowest 20%	35-50%

AR coating dispensed

Median	45-50%
High	80-90%
Low	10-20%

(Practices in the higher range tend to include AR automatically in their lens offerings. The average 60-year-old patient has approximately one-third of the light entering their eyes compared to the average healthy 20-year-old. Then, factor in that lenses without AR coating are losing an additional 8-14% of the light through reflections or type of material. We are not helping the problem of less useful light for older patients. We are exacerbating it.)

Photochromics dispensed

Median	20%
High	30-50%
Low	5-11%

(AR and Photochromics are often packaged together to offer the patients light control technology, which allows more light in when they need it and less light when glare and bright sunlight are a problem. A versatile package—especially for the 50+ club.

Always ask this age group (more than 50 years old) two questions: Do you have trouble reading signs

WHICH LOOKS BETTER, 1 OR 2?

while driving at night? Have you noticed you are more sensitive in bright sunlight?)

Rx sun wear

Median	10%
High	20-30%
Low	2-5%

(In spite of the fact there are more accidents caused by glare than caused by falling asleep at the wheel or driving on the wrong side of the road, these numbers remain low. Also, what a patient wears outside during the day in bright sunlight affects how well she will see at night. Proper filters worn during the day in bright sunlight help with dark adaptation. Patients are not being up-served in this important area.)

Computer lenses

Median	5%
High	15-20%
Low	2-5%

(Another great opportunity for up-serving your patients, young, old and in-between. The key may be in blue light education. Blue emitted from digital devices has been shown to damage the retina. It also suppresses melatonin production which aids in sleep. This produces insomnia which can create problems with concentration, especially for teenagers who spend so many of their waking hours attached to their smart phones. Studies also reveal this can interfere with the hormones which regulate appetite, increasing weight gain.)

By-the-numbers checklist:

There are two major drivers of the fiscal health of your practice.
1. Volume of patients.
2. Revenue per patient.

If you have a low volume of patients, you will need high revenue per patient. If you have low revenue per patient, you will need a high volume of patients.

There are five functions which occur in your office and business every day. You cannot ignore any one of these functions.

- ✓ Sales: do you have a daily sales goal? Does everyone know their part in accomplishing it?
- ✓ Marketing: both internal and external. Internal is critical, because this patient will make a decision in the next hour.
- ✓ Finances: this includes budgetary issues; controlling cost, understanding profit centers.
- ✓ Retention and referrals. This is the function of customer service and everyone is involved in retaining current patients and creating referrals for new patients through up-serving your current patients. Are you asking for and actively seeking referrals?
- ✓ The number one priority of your practice/business is to create and manage the perception of value so you are the Preferred Provider of Choice.

Chapter 15: Up-Serving Communications and Strategies

Have you ever noticed how unfriendly many of our signs are?

>NO PARKING!
>PARKING FOR EYE CLINIC ONLY—VIOLATORS WILL BE TOWED AT THEIR OWN EXPENSE!
>NO SOLICITING!
>NO SKATEBOARDING!
>NO CHECKS!
>NO LOITERING!
>SHOPLIFTERS WILL BE PROSECUTED!

Why not just put a sign that says, "Don't buy anything from us!!"

This section was included to help you with ideas for Up-Serving Communications, Telling the Best Story, the innovative, the unique, the personalized and the fascinating. We will share letters, scripts, factoids and much more. Please free to edit and/or change as best suits your needs and personality.

Remember, your patients do not make up stories about your office, you and your team create the stories they will tell.

Let's turn the mundane into the memorable! Let's ask more questions than "Which Looks Better 1 or 2?" And always be sure your office speaks with ONE VOICE.

Below are some helpful tools to implement up-serving.

Up-serving Letters (edit as you see fit)
Reactivation letter

Dear_____

Our records indicate it has been over three years since your last eye health examination. We are concerned about the health of your vision.

If you have decided to go elsewhere, we will be glad to forward your records.

In the case you have not gone elsewhere and simply overlooked this important health issue, we want to encourage you to contact our office and make an appointment. If you do this within the next 30 days, we are offering a special, "Welcome Back" package.

However, if we do not hear from you in the next thirty days, we will place your name in an inactive file.

Please let us hear from you.

Your name and contact information

- This reactivation letter is a simple reminder to those who have not responded in previous efforts to recall.

WHICH LOOKS BETTER, 1 OR 2?

- Sending just two of these letters per day enables your office to reach more than 40 patients per month.
- The "welcome back" package can be of your choosing. Some use gift cards for local restaurants.
- The "inactive file" does not actually exist, but it sounds like something one would want to avoid!

Letter to Newcomers/New Residents

Dear Mr. & Mrs._____
Welcome to Jackson.

We take pride in being neighborly in Jackson and helpful to new residents. That goes for our office too. We at Family Eye Care would like you to know we are here for you when you need us.

We have enclosed a patient brochure to help acquaint you with our practice and services. You will see it contains a map of our location, office hours and phone numbers. You may also visit our website at www._____.
We accept most major insurances and third-party programs.

Again welcome to Jackson! Please call us if you need our services or have any questions.

Your name and contact information

Tim Fortner

Letter to Local Elementary School Teacher/Principal

Dear_____

As a new school year begins and you are getting to know your students we want to make available to you some important information regarding their vision.

One in four children has an undetected vision problem which can interfere with their learning. Scientists tell us 80% of our learning from birth to age 12 comes from through our vision system.

A child who has an undiagnosed vision problem can have difficulties learning to read, see the blackboard or playing games which require eye-hand coordination. They can become easily frustrated.

They may experience frequent headaches or rub their eyes often.

We have some helpful materials we can make available for your classroom.

These materials are great educational tools as well and will help your students and parents be more aware of potential vision problems.

Please contact our office for this free classroom material.

Your name and contact information

WHICH LOOKS BETTER, 1 OR 2?

Letter for Speaking Opportunities

Dear Lions Club:

As a group who supports healthy sight and worthwhile causes, I wanted to volunteer to speak to your members regarding "Healthy Vision in the 21st Century."

There is a rising concern about healthy vision in America as we have become an aging population. Living longer and working longer in this digital age presents challenges health-wise, not the least of which is healthy vision.

-I have a short video, some very timely data, as well as handouts and websites where one may get additional information.

As a Doctor of Optometry and member of both national and local associations, I have developed a short 20-minute presentation, which is both entertaining and educational.

I will call you later to inquire about your interest and possible dates.

Your name and contact information

Letter to Established Patient

Dear Mrs. Fortner (Gina)

It was a pleasure seeing you in our office the other day. I could not help but notice as I was reviewing your records; you and your family have been patients of our office for 12 years!

The purpose of this letter is just to say, "Thank-you!" My team and I would like to express our gratitude for you continued trust in our ability to maintain your vision health. Providing you and your family with lifelong healthy vision is our main goal.

It is a pleasure to have loyal patients and I wanted you to know we value our longstanding relationship.

As a token of our appreciation I have enclosed_____.

Your name and contact information

Letter to Pharmacists

Dear_____

Several of our patients tell us they use your services. We ask all our patients to list their current medications. Many mention your name personally as their pharmacist.

As a growing practice, we wanted you to know that we are able to accommodate any clients of yours who are

WHICH LOOKS BETTER, 1 OR 2?

in need of our service. We not only write Rx's—we also recommend certain vitamins and over the counter products. I have enclosed a list of those things we recommend.

I have enclosed a patient brochure that describes our services. You can also visit our website at www._____
Give us a call if we might be of service to you and your clients.
Your name and contact information

Letter to Health Club or Spa

Dear_____

Several of our patients tell us they use your services and facilities.

As a growing practice, we want you to know we are able to accommodate any of your clients who are in need of our professional services. We have produced a patient brochure to help answer questions about our practice.

Like you, we work with people's life style to enhance their performance on the job as well as in sports or hobbies. We provide sun wear for protection from glare, as well as safety eyewear to protect one in sports—from handball and racquet ball to basketball.

I have enclosed several copies of information for protecting one's eyesight when involved in such activities.

For additional information or more copies feel free to contact us. We also have a quarterly newsletter.

Your name and contact information

Conversational Education

Facts about vision and the eye can provide interesting information and make the best story even more memorable. And the information adds to your credibility and to the patient's appreciation of the importance of healthy sight counseling.

Remember our goal is to turn the mundane into the memorable. For instance, there is nothing more routine in the clinical process than a blood pressure check. Imagine this scenario as you begin the process and the tech begins the process using a style we call "conversational education."

> *"Mrs. Irvine, I will be performing an auto refraction at this point plus checking your blood pressure. Many people do not realize blood pressure can impact their vision. Do you have any idea how extensive our blood vessel network is? By this I mean if we took all of your blood vessels out of your body and laid them end to end—how far do you think they would reach? I have no idea! Would you believe, laid end to end, they reach 60,000 miles?!"*

WHICH LOOKS BETTER, 1 OR 2?

Watch the raised eyebrows. Observe the shaking of the head in wonder. You have done it. You have fascinated your patient with information about themselves which they did not know that they needed to know. Don't stop—here comes the follow-up:

> *"And unfortunately when we gain one pound of fat, just sixteen ounces of fat, not muscle, your body has to produce another 7 miles of blood vessels just to service that one pound!"*

Think about how their conversation about their eye exam might go tonight when asked about it!! Some other interesting facts to share:

- The eyes blink an average of four million times per year (4,000,000). So if the average time between visits is 2.3 years, your patient had blinked more than ten million times since their last exam. Here is what I would want to know of this patient: "Where in the blink have you been?"
- The eye is approximately the size of a ping pong ball that contains more than two million working parts.
- The average healthy 20-year-old eye allows up to three times as much light than the average 60-year-old.
- During the course of a day, scientists estimate your eyes as they adjust to different types of lighting conditions and focal distances, will expend the same amount of energy

proportionately your leg muscles would if you walked fifty miles.
- Vision requires reflected light. There is no information in direct light source—be it the sun, a lamp or any direct light source.
- Light travels at 186,282 miles per second. In the snap of your fingers it has encircled the earth 7.5 times. There is nothing faster than the speed of light. It is the main component of Einstein's Theory of Relativity. Einstein came to a point in his career where he said he would do nothing but study the phenomena of light. There is nothing like it—it has no mass and no charge.
- When light enters the eye the process of vision begins. The eye and its components change the speed of light, the direction of light as it refracts it and the amount of light.
- The light and the information it carries are focused on the back of the eye, the retina, which is brain tissue. There are more than 130 million photoreceptor cells convert the light into electrical-chemical impulses sent via the optic nerve to the brain to give us our perception of the world around us.
- This transforming process is one of the highest metabolic activities in the human body. In fact the eye and the brain which make up only 2% of your total body weight consume 25% of your nutrition.

WHICH LOOKS BETTER, 1 OR 2?

- Every time you blink, your eyes use 200 muscles. And women, on average blink twice as much as men.
- The fluid in your eyes changes every 15 minutes during the day. What a self-contained, self-healing, self-cleaning phenomena! No wonder Charles Darwin said the human eye made him doubt his own theory of evolution.
- We are solar-powered creatures; light wakes us up in the morning. It is like our body's alarm clock. The human eyes perceive this illumination and send a signal to the brain to wake up.
- The human body has more than 100 alarms related to light which regulate our sleep patterns, temperature, energy, mood, mental acuteness, muscular speed and accuracy, endurance, sexual appetite, hunger and thirst, and indeed our overall well-being and health are related to light and/or the absence of it.
- When direct light strikes an object, three things happen (or a combination of these three): light is reflected; refracted (passes through); or absorbed. If absorbed, light creates energy.
- Vision is very much a high brain activity and there are more than 32 different visual processing centers located in the brain.
- There are four types of glare: distracting glare—caused by reflections off of uncoated

lenses. Disarming glare—glare which occurs when going from indoor lighting to outdoor lighting, bright sunlight between 3,000 and 10,000 lumens, causing ocular discomfort, squinting, reduced contrast and slower dark adaptation. Disabling glare—more than 10,000 lumens and causing ocular discomfort, reduced contrast, slower dark adaptation and blocked vision. Fourth type of glare—blinding glare which is reflected light that blocks vision, causes vision discomfort, reduced contrast and inhibits night vision.

- The automobile insurance industry reports some type of glare is involved in one-third of most accidents. Statistics tell us there are more accidents caused by glare than falling asleep at the wheel or driving in the wrong direction. *This is why controlling light in various condition is so important and in some cases in life threatening conditions.*
- The brain has 100 billion neurons with each having the ability to make up to 10,000 connections. This number is one (1) quadrillion: 1,000,000,000,000,000. During an average day, these one quadrillion connections send 8.6 quadrillion electronic messages across the electronic grid of the brain in fractions of seconds. When we take the 50 billion cell phone calls, 17 billion text messages and 300 billion emails, the seven billion people on earth send each day—they

come to be only 1/200th of 1% of what goes in the human brain per day! Absolutely amazing! And the majority of information coming from the five senses is from our eyes, the human vision system. Surely it is worth more than the current 24 cents per day we are spending on vision care!

Well-Thought-Out Answers

"Can I have my Rx and PD?"

Many have already received this request and this is not going away. You may have also noticed more of your patients taking photos of your frames with their smart phones.

Welcome to the 21st century shopper. A smart, internet savvy consumer who aided by a world of information via their smart phone has become better at buying than most of us are selling.

But remember, we are replacing the word "selling" with up-serving.

Now about that request: Say, "No, we do NOT have to provide the PD, only the Rx." And you will probably never see that patient and/or their family members again.

Here is the answer: *"Yes and to do so, we charge a fee ($25-40) for our verification and adjustment program, something the internet cannot do. This will allow you to bring you glasses back to us so we can verify the Rx is correct and meets ANSI industry standards of acceptance. We can provide you an actual read out of your lenses' prescription as well* *if it meets the standards of what was prescribed. This way, we can be sure you are receiving the correct Rx for which you were prescribed. The adjustment is to make sure not only that you are comfortable, but seeing through the optical centers as they were designed to perform. If your lenses do not meet the standards, we will help you send them back with the documented information as to why these should be remade or your money refunded."*

Always find a way to say, "Yes, and..."

The proactive measure is to put together a Patient Services Agreement. This lists all the services you provide—which includes your fees. It will also be a way of comparison to reveal all the things not provided when purchasing vision correction online. These services can make all the difference in whether a patient can see at their best.

"What do I get with my plan?"

Answer: "Anything you want!"

It's critical to think of the patient's plan as the floor, not the ceiling! Talk to them in terms of the discount their plan offers, not what their plan "covers."

So the full answer to, "What do I get with my plan?" is, *"Anything you want! We have a prescription plan that addresses your key vision issues. Your plan provides a nice discount: instead of the $400 another patient would pay, your cost is $275 for a pair of everyday glasses with photochromic lenses and anti-glare, and a pair of computer glasses. You'll be more*

WHICH LOOKS BETTER, 1 OR 2?

comfortable and protected during all your normal activities!"

Warranties and Guarantees

Many top practices post something like this: Seven Reasons Why to Get Your Eyeglasses Here!

1. Two year warranty on all frames. If for any reason (except loss) you need your frames repaired or replaced, we will do it at no charge for two years from the date of purchase.
2. Warranty on lenses with scratch coating and specialty coatings (AR Coating) are also guaranteed for two years from purchase. (Limited to same Rx.)
3. Wide selection of frames, including budget selections plus our 14-day Free Exchange Progam.*
4. Knowledgeable, courteous staff including experienced, trained opticians.
5. Latest technology in High-definition Lenses. See our lens app station.
6. Guaranteed satisfaction with your RX.
7. Highest quality service, available in a pleasant, unhurried atmosphere.

*14-day Free Exchange Program: If for any reason you do not like your new glasses in the first 14-days after being fitted, we will exchange them FREE for another in the same price range.

This may sound like you are asking for trouble, but Best Practices who have implemented this believe when you reduce the risk, you increase the interest.

Up-serving to Overcome Price Objections

There are four proven methods for overcoming price objections. These include: cost over time; relative value; separate the difference; and top down dispensing.

It is also necessary for your team in the dispensary to be familiar with insurance and provider programs and what they provide. Personal testimony is always powerful when your team member can tell the patient, "This is what I choose to wear." Strong warranties and guarantees reduce risk and increase interest.

You may also find certain employees work better with certain type of patients, particularly children or elderly. Others may be better advocates for certain products because they wear them: i.e., photochromics, computer lenses, polarized sun-wear, or AR coating.

Always begin by telling the patient, your goal at this point is to educate them about all which will serve to restore, maintain and enhance their vision

1. <u>Costs over time</u>: The average person wears their glasses for 2.3 years. This is close enough to 1,000 days that to figure costs per day for usage just move the decimal place over 3 places. Example: eyeglasses cost $400. Cost per day: 40 cents. Always say, what can you get for 40 cents a day that you use 14 hours per day, seven days per week? If you paid $400 for a suit, and wore it every day for 14 hours for one thousand days, would you not

consider it to be a great value? And, furthermore, what if you lost a button, got a tear in the material and could return to the seller and they would make the repairs at no cost? Then, consider what their glasses do for them and help them to do all day long and into the night. For most people they are the last thing they took off last night and the first thing they put on in the morning. What can you get for 40 cents that does this much for you? You cannot buy a stamp, a coke, a candy bar or a pack of gum for 40 cents per day. But we can provide patients with something that enhances their quality of life and enables them to perform tasks which you could not without your glasses. Price is what you pay—value is what you get. We provide what is one of the most necessary items to function properly for extremely daily low costs. What a value!

2. <u>Relative Value</u>: This strategy gets the person to think about what else they spend their money on and what they get for it. Common comparison is eating out, dining at your favorite restaurant. Eating at an Olive Garden, Long Horn, Out Back, etc. is very popular, as they are filled most every night. Not uncommon for a couple eating here and enjoying all the amenities, cocktails, wine with their meal, dessert and coffee plus gratuity, to spend a $100. An enjoyable evening, and we understand their desire for such

entertainment. But as you pass by those empty plates, you realize for the cost of their meal—they could have had AR coating on their lenses which they do not, which is why they are having trouble reading their bill in the low light. AR coating, the cost of one evenings' dining out experience, could provide them with enhanced vision and enjoyment for the next 2.3 years. After all, where will this food be in 24 hours?

3. <u>Separate the difference</u>: Mrs. Irvine is a regular patient who regularly spends $375 on her eyeglasses, always selecting some fashionable new frames or styles to add to her wardrobe. She has trouble reading signs at night and at her age would benefit from adding AR coating. This brings the price of her eyewear up to $475. But this is not a $475 decision—this is a $100 decision. She had already budgeted in her mind to spend her usual $375, so the decision is about spending $100 for something which will benefit her 14 hours per day for the next 1,000 days.

4. <u>Top down dispensing</u> is a very effective method in today's market of multiple lens applications and benefits. Many refer to a multiple pair solution as a Program or Plan. This is our Baby Boomer Program—perfect for the conditions occurring as a result of the natural aging process. Always ask this age group two questions: Are you having trouble

WHICH LOOKS BETTER, 1 OR 2?

reading signs at night when driving? Have you noticed you are more sensitive in bright sunlight? We know that, as one ages, he or she will have difficulties with small print, low light, dark adaptation, night vision and bright sunlight. Offer this patient a light control program to solve the problem. This involves the use of two popular lens enhancements: AR coating and Photochromics. These two lens apps are a perfect pair for letting in more light when the patient needs it and filtering bright sunlight instantly to provide comfort in bright sunlight. This is one of the most versatile single pair of primary eye wear you can provide. Also includes UV filter and, recently also, blue light filter. Offer a discount when purchasing this program or plan. (This plan can also include a pair of polarized sunwear and computer lenses.)

Once the patient is educated about the choices, insurance and discount are applied. If the patient says this is more than I can afford at this time. Then you can offer some suggestions for alternatives: a simple lay-away plan; or the use of popular no-interest programs provided by such providers as Care Credit, a GE company used by health care professional every day in this world of higher deductibles and changes in insurance contributions.

But always work with the customer's budget to provide the best benefits for their budget.

Tim Fortner

For example: Offering a patient an AR coated primary pair of High-definition lenses, plus a pair of prescription polarized sun-wear might be more than they can afford. The industry data shows the average practice fits only 10% of their patients with polarized prescription eyewear, with only 20% plus being dispensed in those recognized as being in the tops in their profession. So 80-90% of the patients do not opt for polarized sun wear which means this is a great opportunity for a top-down situation.

Dispenser: *"We understand budget issues and here is what we can do to solve these problems. Let's get the AR plus photochromics, which will give you the light filtering feature in bright sunlight and protect you from glare and preserve your night vision. Photochromics work well with AR coating and you will still have the benefit of the indoor clarity as well as driving at night. With your new frame we can also provide a polarized driving clip for day time driving. This provides you the most versatile pair of glasses we can design."* (Notice you have gone from the greater price to the lesser price, while still balancing the budget with the benefits, a great fall back strategy, while saving your patient money.)

Consider having a lens demonstration center with demonstration lenses and brochures. Refer to this as your LENS APP STATION. Complete with UV demonstrator for photochromics (contact Transition Lenses); a polarized sun lens demo; AR demo kit and a side by side comparison of high index lenses.

WHICH LOOKS BETTER, 1 OR 2?

The information and education and hands on demonstrations are what the consumer cannot get online. In a world where anyone can find anything with a few keystrokes on their computers, many think this is the death of the salesman. No, the salesman has been resurrected as teacher, educator and expert who can enlighten one's self-interest by providing personalized health care. Involving the patient in the process is key; after all it is their eyesight at stake.

Learn how to ask good questions. Being able to ask good questions is equally as important as having good well-thought-out answers to frequently asked questions.

Helping your patients find the right answers for their best vision and best health is accomplished by empathizing, nurturing and guiding the patient through the process.

Up-serving and Enlightened Self-Interest

Self-interest is a very basic human instinct.

We have a natural barrier of self-preservation—self-interest which guards against injury, harm or loss which includes financial loss. No one wants to buy something they do not need or pay more for something than is needed. There is a natural barrier between buyer and seller which guards against "up-selling." And now we have a buyer who is better at buying than sellers are at selling, which means the barrier we must break through has gotten even tougher.

Tim Fortner

How do we get past this barrier? We enlighten their self-interest by telling them something they didn't know about themselves, something they need to know to improve the quality of their life. *So we align with their self-interest, we don't fight against it!*

First you have to get their attention. You can't make someone listen. You can entice, inspire, stimulate or fascinate. Affluence creates boredom and, when you add the addiction we have to our ever-present smart phones, we have a society and culture which have not only become a near point society, but also one afflicted with mass Attention Deficit Disorder.

Once you get someone's attention, you can leverage their "enlightened self-interest"--in this case, their interest in their vision.

How interested are people in their vision/eyesight? A survey done by the American Foundation for Blindness asked the question: What is your greatest health fear as most negatively impacting your quality of life? The answer was very revealing. Two answers tied for the number one answer: Being paralyzed and going blind. Heart attacks, cancer, strokes and all types of serious illness were further down the list of fears. The survey states the obvious: loss of sight, going blind is a great fear. In other words, self-interest is very high! Leverage this high level of self-interest with conversational education.

Remember: today's consumers like the innovative, personalized and fascinating. Let's give

WHICH LOOKS BETTER, 1 OR 2?

them something to talk about! Let's change the conversation they will have tonight about their eye examination you and your team provided today.

UP-SERVING TO CREATE PERSONAL SERVICE

Steve Jobs, the visionary founder of Apple once said: "It's not the customer's job to know what they need." It is your job. Engaging with patients will help you create personal service, the memorable sort of experience that will keep them loyal to your practice.

We like to talk about "RPM"—providing the best RESULTS for the most PATIENTS by the best possible MEANS. RPM by definition revolves around the patient—it's the perfect opportunity to demonstrate your passion for helping patients enjoy their best possible vision for as long as possible.

Another acronym we like is K.E.E.P. It's another way to focus your office on creating personal service through up-serving.

- **Knowledge**—yours and your team's clinical and product knowledge combined with knowledge about your patient, their lifestyle, their family. Use your patient update profile to keep this current. Make notes.

- **Enlightening** Education-education is powerful. But it must be fascinating, personal and not boring. If you find yourself saying the same things to all your patients, you're probably not being very fascinating; you're not providing personal service!

- **Evaluation** and Engagement—involve the patient in an honest evaluation of what the solutions you are recommending will do for their vision and lifestyle. Engage them in the decision process.

- **Positive** conversation—his will involve what solutions are more important; if three pairs are recommended—and patient can only afford two of them—which should be the priorities. Balance the benefits with the budget and offer financial opportunities

EPILOGUE

Every generation of eye care professionals has had to deal with challenges, new technology, competition, fads and trends. What we have shared is what Best Practices tell us they have found as the answer to vision care in the 21st century. The answer for my daughter was the same as it was for my brother and father before them. The answer was there all the time—when they raised their hands and pledged to do the following:

> "I will fully and honestly advise my patients of all which may *serve* to restore, maintain or enhance their vision and general health."
> (Optometric Oath)

This oath applies to all of us who provide vision care.

The answer is found in the simple word—**Serve.** Serve is defined as, "To perform duties or service for another person." The goal of such service is to improve the quality of the other person's life.

To do this service must be: personal and purposeful.

Up-serving is how one makes service personal and purposeful. It is more than a strategy; it is a philosophy and attitude. It is the opposite of upselling and it is powerful. It turns the mundane into memorable and the facts into personal, purposeful and fascinating.

It is not only having the best story to tell. It is about becoming the best storytellers.

It has been my honor and a pleasure to spend time with you and learn from every one of you.

God bless you for all you do each day to help people enjoy the incredible gift of sight!

-Tim

About the Author

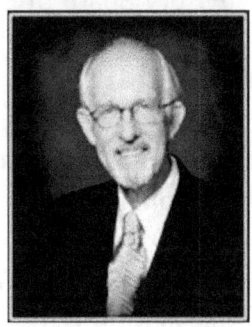

Tim has spent almost 50 years in the optical industry. His experience includes:
- Vice President of Muller Optical and Progressive Lens Lab
- President of Creative Concepts
- Manager of Training and Education, Transitions Optical
- Chief of Ophthalmic Services and Adjunct Professor, Southern College of Optometry
- Manager of Trade Development for North America, Transitions Optical
- CEO and Founder of Fortner Consulting Group
- Frequent contributor to professional journals

Mr. Fortner has been a popular lecturer in the USA, Canada and abroad. He is known for his storytelling and innovative, research-driven insight into patient behavior.

Tim Fortner

Tim has served on:

- National Panel on Presbyopia
- Editorial Advisory Board of Eye Care Business Magazine
- OLA Regional Boards
Awards:
- Varilux Distributor Sales Person of Year
- Two Time Recipient of Transitions Award of Distinction
- Featured Speaker @ International Symposium on Presbyopia in Morocco
- Coauthor of: Making Managed Care Work for You, Published by OLA

Contact Tim @: johntfortner@gmail.com
Tim Fortner, 35 Seventeen Green, Jackson, TN 38305

Visit our website:

https://FortnerConsultingGroup.com for additional information and how to join our blog: The Up-Serving Institute.

Available for Continuing Education both COPE Practice Management; ABO and Para-Optometric approved seminars.

www.ingramcontent.com/pod-product-compliance
Lightning Source LLC
Chambersburg PA
CBHW071439180526
45170CB00001B/383